This Book Belongs To:

_____

My Healthy Selfie!
(Draw yourself here)

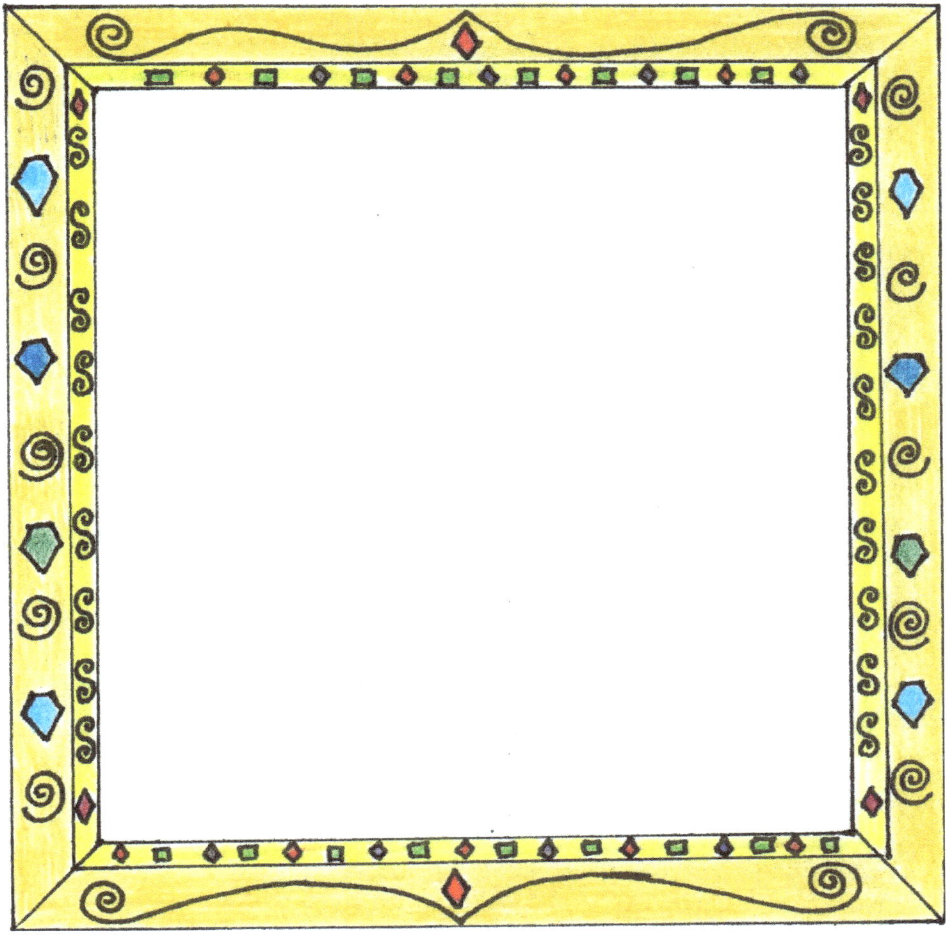

ExtraOrdinary Kids Guide to Health

Dedication

To my two wonderful children (Jessica & Nicholas) who are my inspiration for this book!

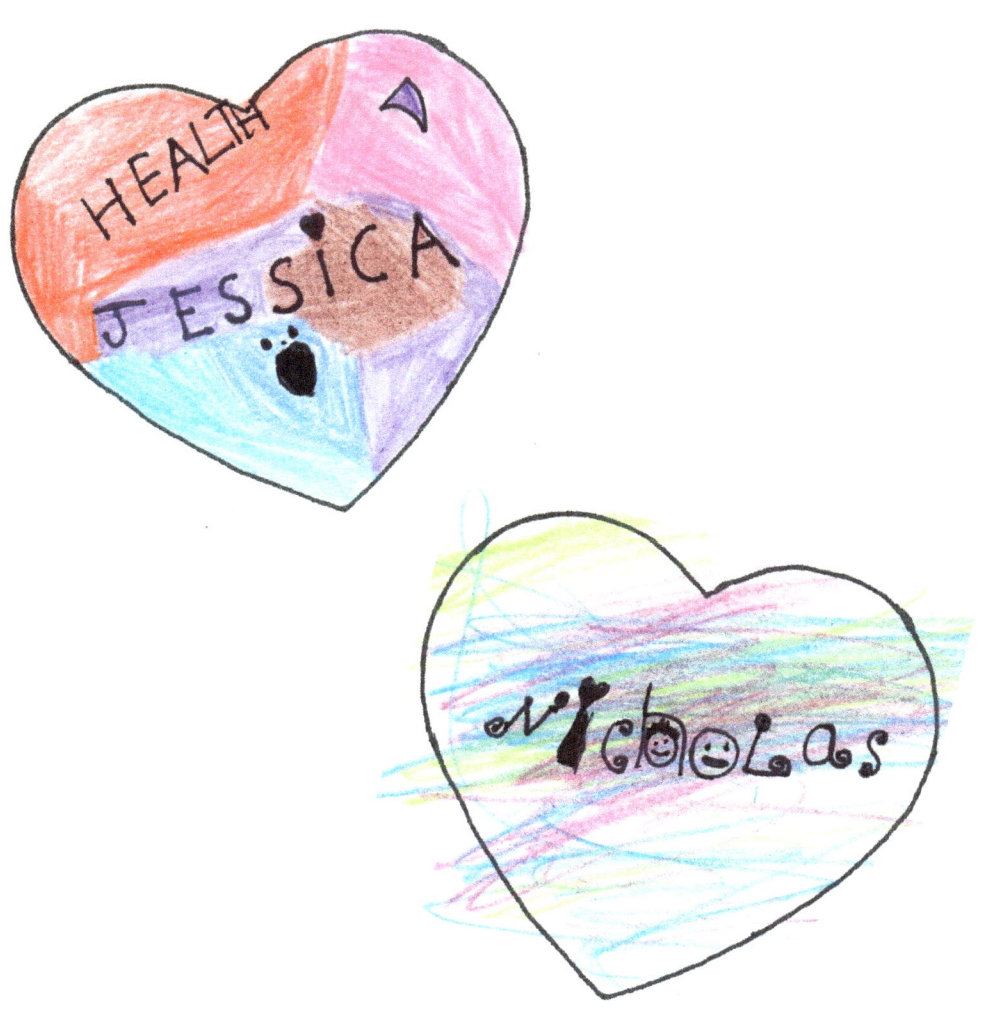

Acknowledgements

I want to thank all those that helped me make this book a reality!

Thank you to Jessica, Sarah Pasemann, Donna Tyson, John and Tara Gloor for reviewing and giving me valuable input.

Thank you to Judy Pasemann and Ryan Arvin for doing a final review.

Thank you God for guiding me along the way.

I am so grateful!
Melanie

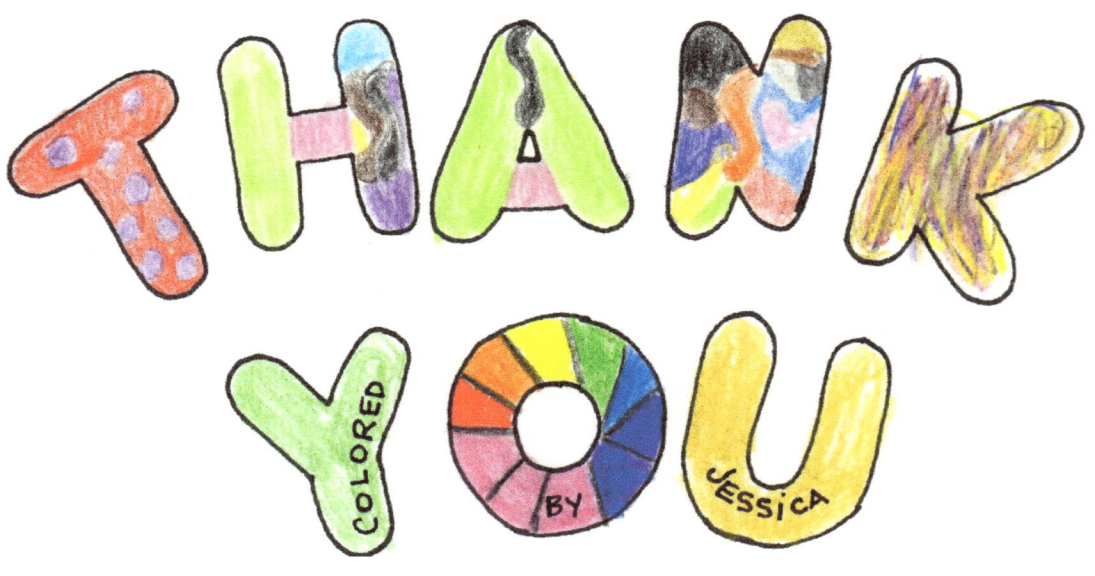

Introduction

This book is written for kids!
It was inspired by kids!
Written & illustrated by a 40 something big kid! 🙂

How to Use

I wrote this book to be a fun guide to learning more about health. There are a variety of topics. Each topic includes a poem and illustration on the left side of the page and then additional information, a challenge, or activity on the right hand side.

My intention is for you to carry it around and use it as a journal and to enjoy the challenges and activities included. Make it a goal to cover one to two topics per week. Take your time to absorb the information and enjoy!

Feel free to get your parents involved as well and share this extraordinary information! In addition, skipping around in the book is okay; no need to go in order.

Bonus: There is a secret code to decode at the end of this book (see page 67)!

(Note: These are my views on what it takes to be healthy.)

Table of Contents

The Eat Good & Exercise Stuff!

Organic/Local

Eat lots of healthy fruit and vegetables;
Food that is organically or locally grown;
Free of fertilizers and pesticides- the bad stuff;
To fuel your body, brain and to grow strong bones!

Steer clear of certain foods,
Such as corn, sugar, and soy;
Most of these crops are genetically modified;
To our bodies and Mother Earth it will certainly destroy!

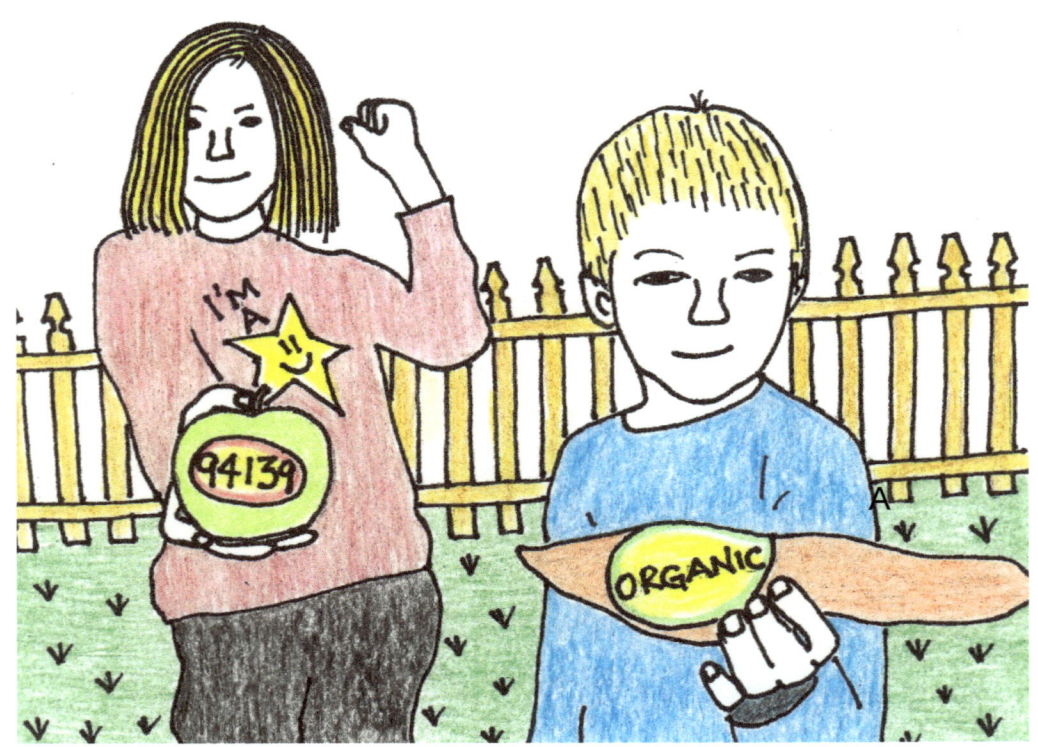

Definitions:

<u>Organic</u>-Organic food:

1) Is produced by farmers who nurture (care for) the land (environment) in which their crops are grown.

2) Organic animal products (meat, eggs, etc.) come from animals that are given no antibiotics or growth hormones (chemicals to make animals grow bigger).

3) Is produced without using most conventional pesticides & fertilizers and does not contain GMOs (see below).

4) Has to be inspected & certified before being labeled 'organic'.

<u>Local</u>-Commonly, "local food" refers to food produced near the consumer and associated with <u>sustainable agriculture</u> (fresh, healthful, and produced in a responsible manner).

<u>Conventional</u>-Food grown typically with using chemical fertilizers & pesticides, antibiotics, growth hormones, and GMOs (see below).

<u>GMO (Genetically Modified Organism)</u>-Genetic modification is the process of forcing genes from one species into another unrelated species. The top three GMO foods are: corn, soy, and canola.

Challenge: Fruits & vegetables are labeled with a number:

5 digit number starting with '9' =Organic
5 digit number starting with '8' =GMO (genetically modified)
3 or 4 digit number =Conventional

At the grocery store, list some organic produce (fruits or vegetables) and the corresponding '9' number:

Example: Bananas_____   __94011____

_____   _____

_____   _____

_____   _____

Vegetables

Your parents are right when they say 'Eat your Veggies';
They should cover half of your plate;
Find the way you like to eat them,
Such as steamed, raw, sautéed, juiced, or baked!

Don't be afraid to try something new,
Maybe radishes, turnips, kale, or green beans;
Choose a colorful variety,
Including reds, yellows and definitely greens!

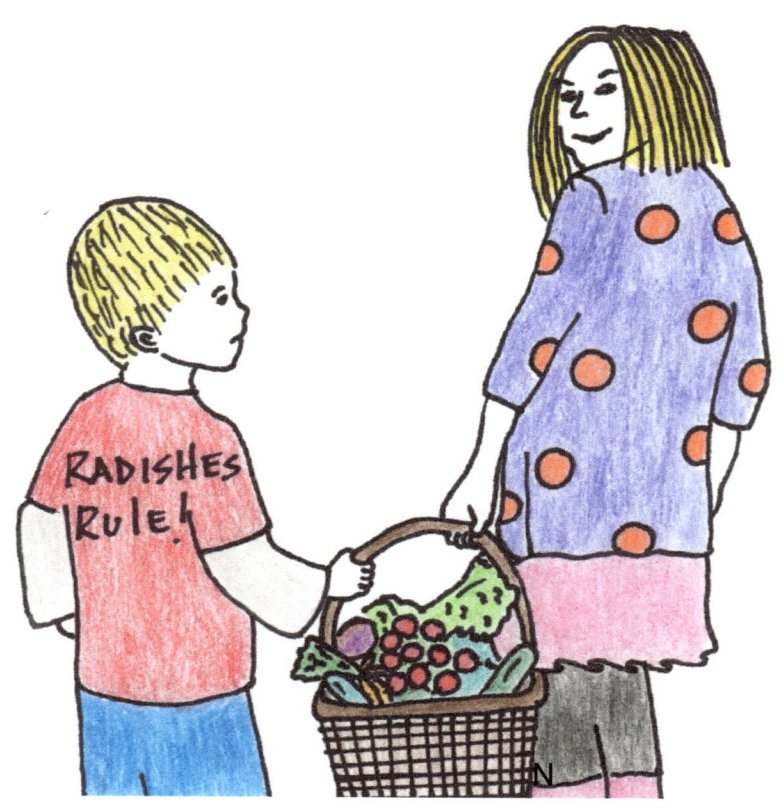

Word Search:

lettuce   broccoli   radish   celery   cucumber
carrot   kale   squash   onion   turnip   spinach
cauliflower   pepper   eggplant   kohlrabi   corn
beets   cabbage   okra   asparagus   artichokes
mushrooms

```
K  O  H  L  R  A  B  I  Z  K  O  O  H  Z  O
F  K  U  S  P  I  N  A  C  H  H  K  R  T  V
Z  E  Z  K  P  C  H  K  A  N  L  E  Y  B  G
R  E  B  M  U  C  U  C  U  T  H  D  R  R  T
R  D  E  R  T  D  E  P  L  N  S  G  E  O  U
Q  C  O  N  I  O  N  H  I  A  I  A  L  C  R
D  O  N  L  B  H  A  P  F  L  D  R  E  C  N
P  R  H  S  A  U  Q  S  L  P  A  K  C  O  I
H  N  T  O  R  R  A  C  O  G  R  O  R  L  P
L  E  T  T  U  C  E  F  W  G  S  H  H  I  K
F  E  G  A  B  B  A  C  E  E  W  A  Q  A  S
R  E  P  P  E  P  Z  I  R  L  Z  I  L  E  T
S  E  K  O  H  C  I  T  R  A  C  E  B  I  E
O  K  M  U  S  H  R  O  O  M  S  N  Y  S  E
Z  C  O  C  U  S  U  G  A  R  A  P  S  A  B
```

Puzzle made at www.puzzle-maker.com

Fruit

When getting your fruit, it is better to eat it,
Rather than to drink it from a cup;
Fruit juice has loads of sugar;
Whole fruit is best- the fiber fills you up!

Fruit still contains sugar,
So enjoy a little and choose a colorful array;
Apples, oranges, lemons & limes are good,
But berries are typically the best for any day!

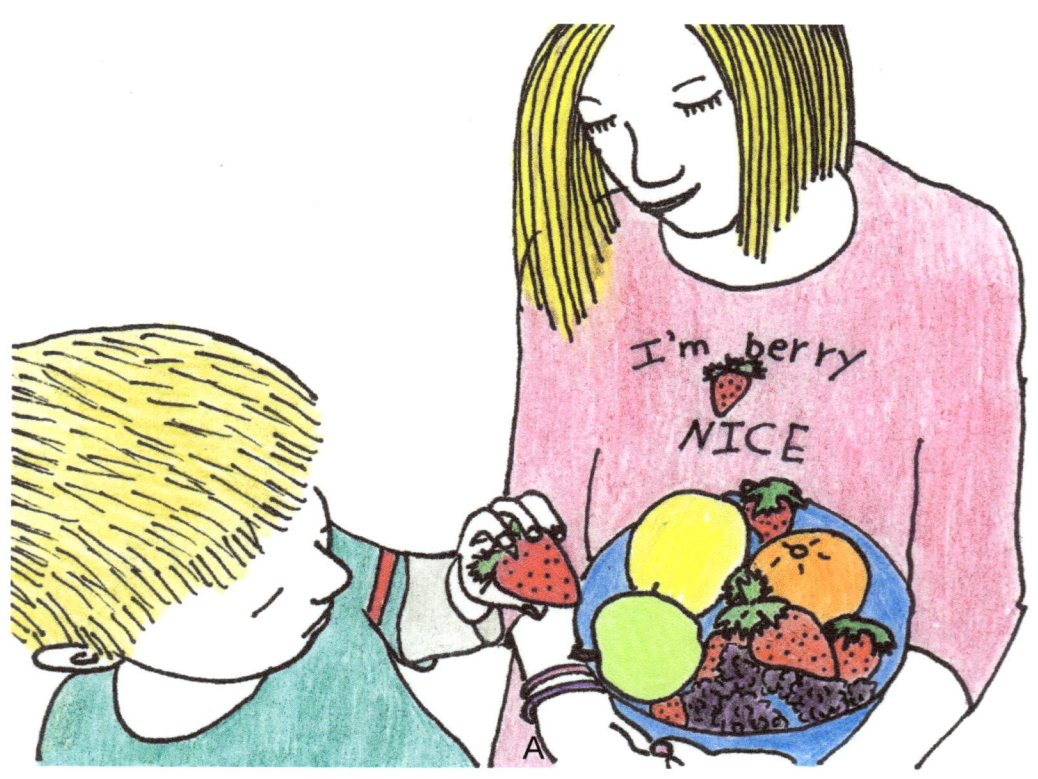

Fact: Did you know that tomatoes and avocados are technically (scientifically) fruits, not vegetables?

Word Search:

pineapple   apple   pear   orange   banana
tangerine   kiwi   lemon   lime   blueberry
strawberry   melon   grape   cherry   apricot   plum
peach

```
F  D  F  C  I  G  A  P  A  Q  G  I  F  Z  I
E  G  Q  H  R  O  P  G  E  I  D  H  A  I  J
L  Q  L  E  G  T  P  E  L  H  L  N  C  N  U
I  I  Y  R  V  Z  L  Y  P  J  A  N  M  J  G
M  Q  A  R  T  E  E  N  P  N  O  H  F  S  I
E  P  D  Y  Y  K  M  P  A  L  N  Q  O  T  B
E  I  M  Z  R  N  V  B  E  J  O  T  R  R  K
F  V  L  U  R  J  T  M  N  N  M  O  A  A  V
C  H  C  A  E  P  Z  F  I  T  E  C  N  W  E
P  L  N  J  B  C  O  Y  P  Y  L  I  G  B  I
T  A  N  G  E  R  I  N  E  X  D  R  E  E  H
H  T  N  I  U  A  I  W  I  K  W  P  L  R  Y
L  N  R  F  L  P  L  U  M  W  M  A  P  R  Q
A  P  S  J  B  H  L  G  T  Y  S  N  Y  Y  R
U  M  T  F  I  F  V  P  E  A  R  H  D  V  I
```

Water

Drink water throughout the day,
To stay hydrated and healthy;
No sodas please-
They are full of chemical additives and are very sugary!

Consume the cleanest water as possible,
Preferably filtered or from wells;
Our bodies are about 60% water,
So drink to refuel your cells!

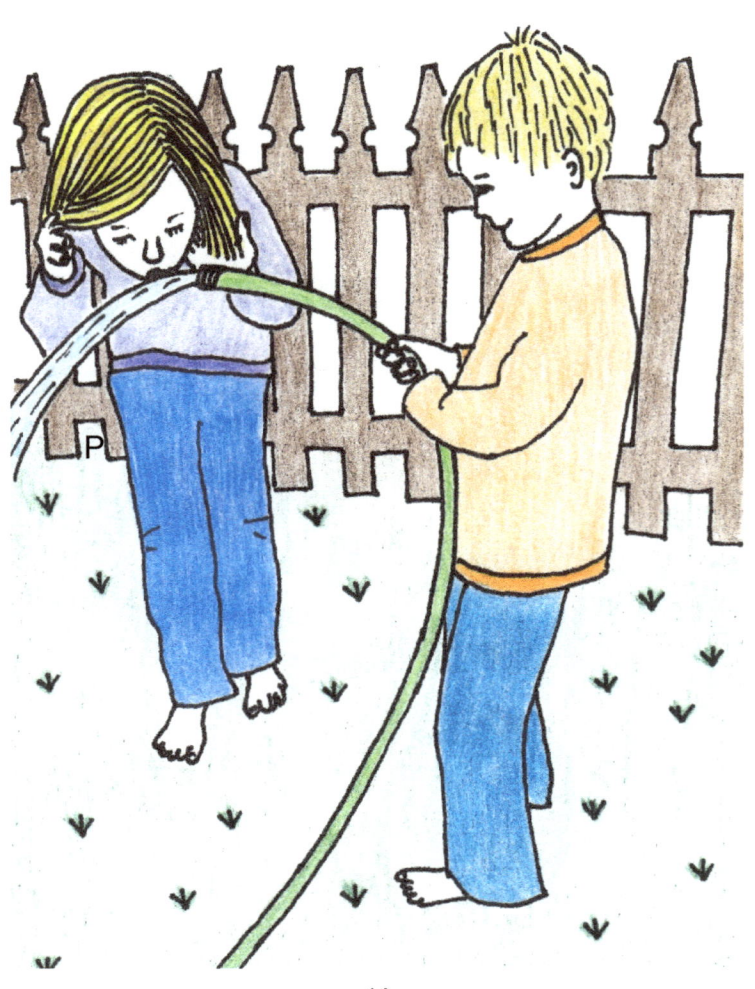

Water Facts:
1) Water is made up of two elements, **hydrogen** and **oxygen**. Its chemical formula is H_2O.
2) The existence of water is essential for life on Earth.
3) Water has three different states: liquid, solid and gas.
4) The word water usually refers to water in its liquid state. The solid state of water is known as ice while the gas state of water is known as steam or water vapor.
5) Water covers around 70% of the Earth's surface.

Challenge:
Drink only water for one week. A rough rule of thumb is to drink about 67% of your body weight in ounces per day; adding extra for exercise or hotter days.

What is 67% of your body weight? _____ ounces/day.
(Example: Weight is 90 pounds. 90 x .67 = approximately 60 ounces.)

What drinks did you replace with water?

_____

_____

_____

_____

_____

Sugar

It is best to limit sugar;
Use it for an occasional treat;
Opt for better, natural alternatives like honey;
If wanting something sweet to eat!

Be aware and on guard;
Sugar is hidden in lots of food;
It makes you feel happy and then sad;
It really affects your mood!

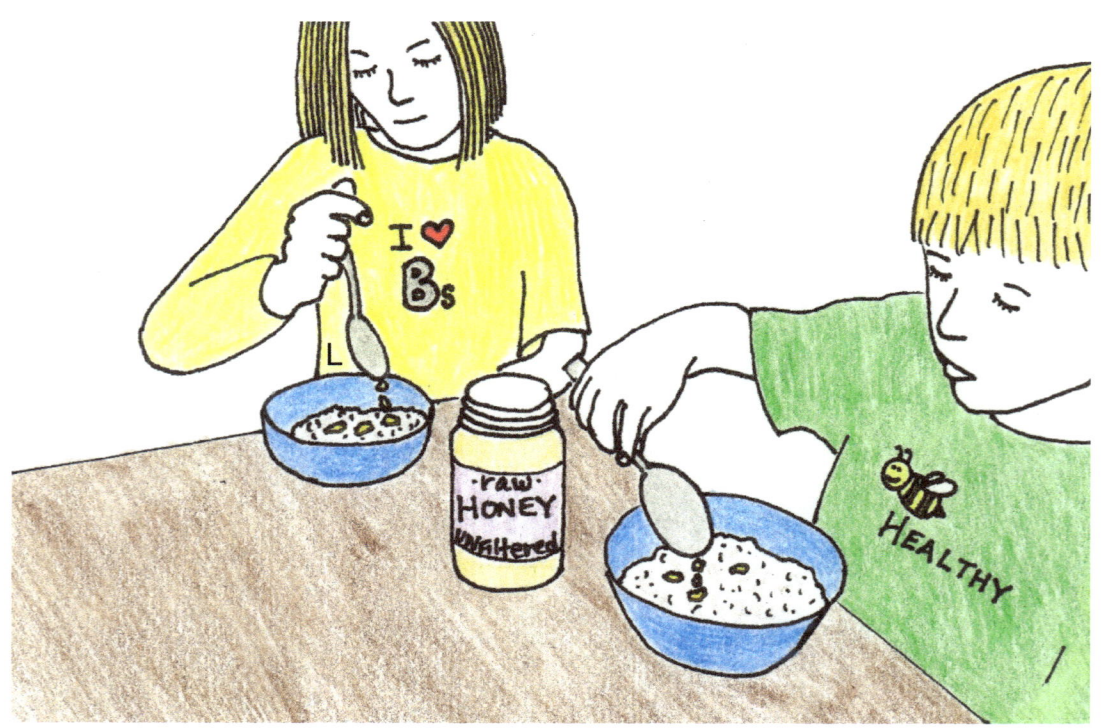

Sugar News:

1) Sugar is addictive. This is the condition of wanting more and more of something (substance, thing, or activity); typically to the point of being harmful in one way or another.

2) Some better, natural sugar alternatives: Honey, Maple Syrup, Molasses, and Dates.

3) Sugar-free foods are not good. That typically means they include artificial (fake) sweeteners which are manufactured chemicals.

4) It is best to limit or avoid added sugars found in most packaged food and beverages. Some examples of common items with high sugar content per serving:

(Note: 1 sugar cube (▢) = about 1 teaspoon of sugar)

Item	Serving Size	Estimated Amount of Sugar	Figure out the # of Teaspoons
Soda	12 oz (1 can)	▢▢ ▢ ▢▢ ▢▢ ▢▢	_____
Apple Juice	8 oz (1 cup)	▢▢ ▢ ▢▢ ▢	_____
Orange Juice	8 oz (1 cup)	▢▢ ▢ ▢▢	_____
Raisins	~handful (1/4 cup)	▢▢ ▢ ▢▢ ▢	_____

Challenge:

At the grocery store, look up the sugar content of one serving of your favorite sweet treat.

Your Favorite Sweet Treat: _____.

The sugar content: _____ per serving.
(Note: Look on the nutrition label under 'Sugars')

Nutrition Labels (Ingredients)

Learn to read nutrition labels,
To know what it is that you eat;
Choose food with less than five items;
Better yet- one ingredient is simple and complete!

Make sure what you eat you can pronounce,
And that the food is real;
No artificial flavorings or colors;
FD&C Blue No. 1 and Red No. 40 are not the best deal!

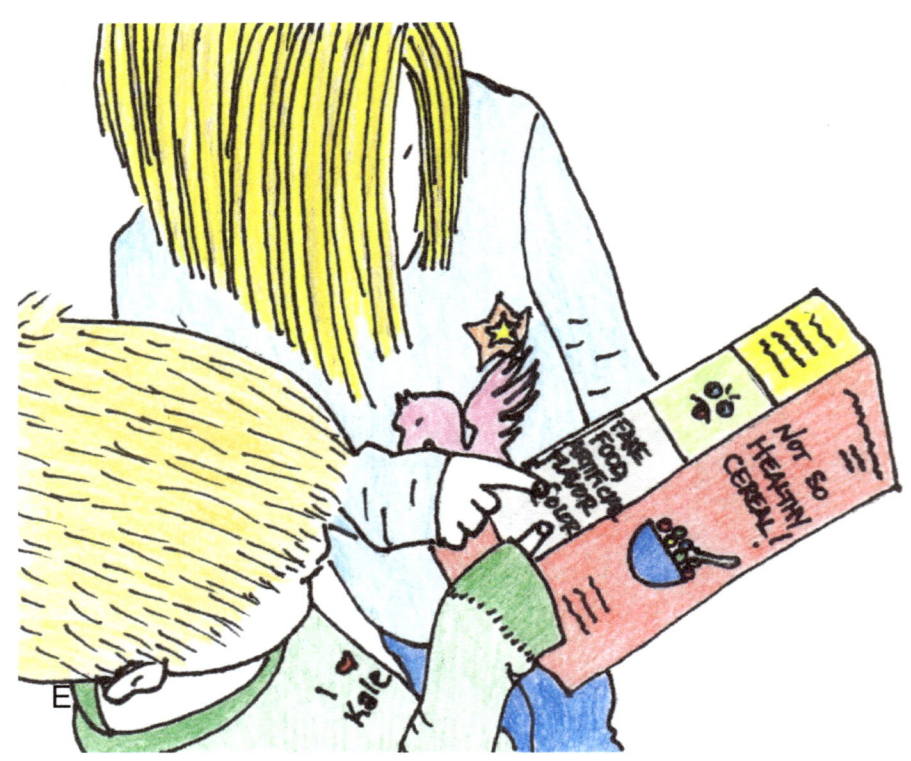

Challenge:

From the nutrition label below, list items that you cannot pronounce. In addition, list items appearing to be artificial (fake) or that do not seem to be real food (i.e. does not appear to grow on a bush or tree!).

Ingredients: Enriched Corn Meal (Corn Meal, Ferrous Sulfate, Niacin, Thiamin Mononitrate, Riboflavin, and Folic Acid), Vegetable Oil (Corn, Canola, and/or Sunflower Oil), Cheese Seasoning (Whey, Cheddar Cheese [Milk, Cheese Cultures, Salt, Enzymes], Canola Oil, Maltodextrin [Made From Corn], Salt, Whey Protein Concentrate, Monosodium Glutamate, Natural and Artificial Flavors, Lactic Acid, Citric Acid, Artificial Color [Yellow 6]), and Salt.
CONTAINS MILK INGREDIENTS.
(Note: Ingredients obtained directly from the bag)

Questionable Ingredients:

_____

_____

_____

_____

_____

_____

_____

Can you guess what food this is? _____

(Answer on page 68)

Mindful Eating

It is best to sit down to eat without distractions;
Don't eat 'on the run' or 'on the go';
Chew your food calmly and thoroughly;
Take your time and eat slow!

Don't eat in front of the TV,
As this makes you consume more; not less.
Be mindful of what you are eating;
The food will be more enjoyable and easier to digest!

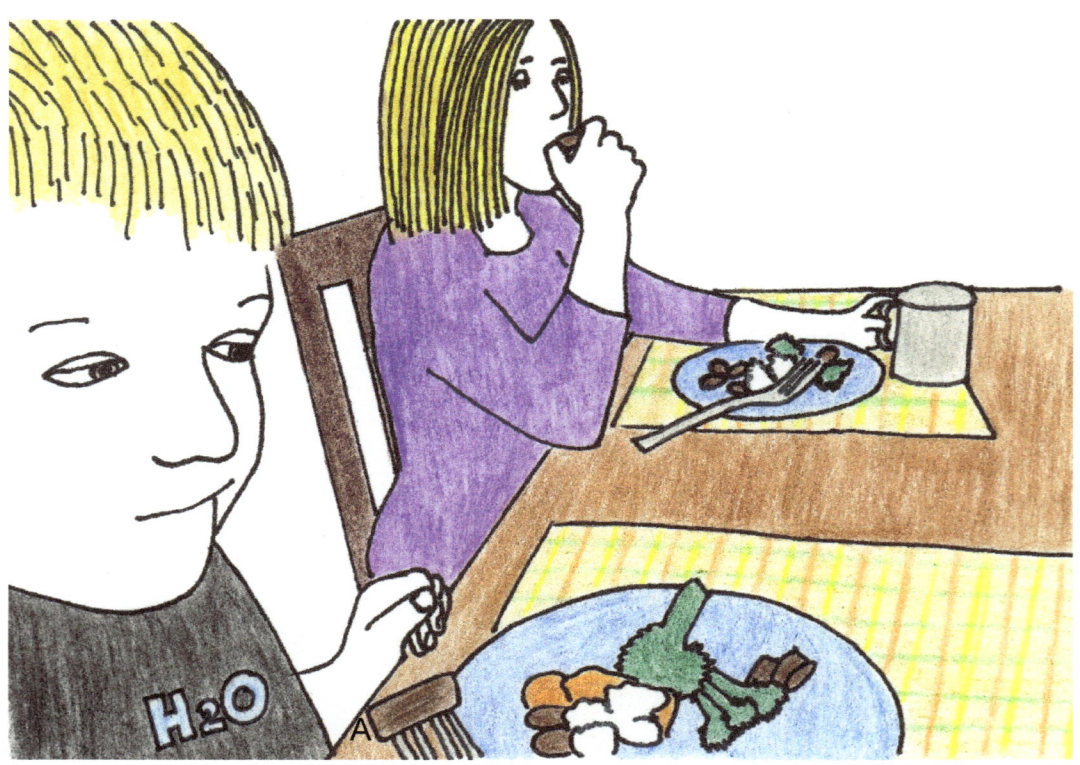

Definition:

Mindful Eating-includes the practice of these principles:
1) Eating with the intention (purpose) to eat. Eating because you are hungry, not because the food is just there.
2) Attention to what you are eating. The textures, flavors, smells, and how it looks.
3) Paying attention to your body's signals: What do you actually want to eat? Are you full? Are you still enjoying the food?
4) Chewing thoroughly and eating slowly.
5) Eating without distractions such as TV, computer, etc.

True (T)/False (F)? (answers on page 68):
1) It is best to eat while watching a movie?   T/F
2) When you are bored, it is best to grab a snack?   T/F
3) It is best to eat because you are hungry?   T/F
4) Chewing your food a lot is a waste of time?   T/F
5) Eating until you're comfortably full is a good rule? T/F

Challenge:
Practice mindful eating.

Track any differences you noticed after eating mindfully:

_____

_____

_____

_____

Macronutrients

It is good to eat well balanced meals,
A combination of fats, carbohydrates, and proteins;
These are called macronutrients;
Essential for your health and well-being!

Some sources of protein include nuts, seeds, and meat;
While olives and avocados are good fats to eat;
For carbs- limit the rice, pasta, and breads;
Opt for the starchy vegetable kind instead!

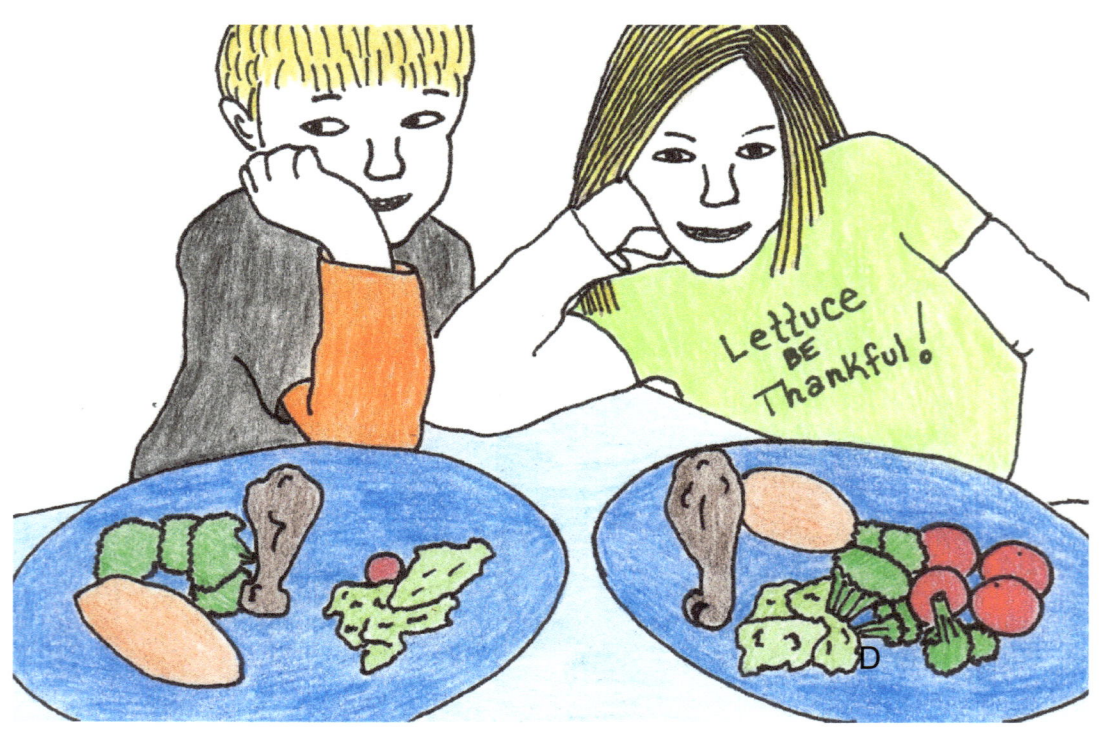

Crossword:

Macronutrients

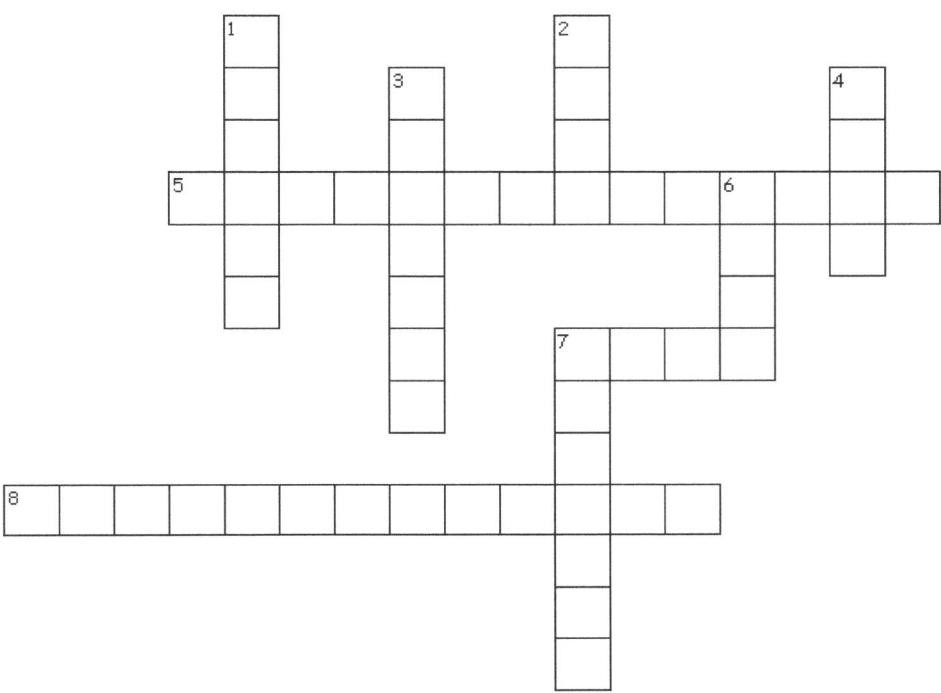

Across

5. Fats, Proteins, and Carbohydrates.
7. A starchy vegetable based carbohydrate found in pods.
8. Its primary job is to fuel the body with energy.

Down

1. A good source of carbohydrates (a starchy vegetable): Sweet _____.
2. An animal food source that provides a good amount of protein.
3. A good fat source that has a green skin.
4. This macronutrient is the major storage form of energy in the body.
6. A good source of protein provided by chickens.
7. Builds, maintains, and replaces the tissues in your body.

Words to choose from: peas, avocado, macronutrients, protein, fats, carbohydrates, potato, meat, eggs

Exercise

Make sure to get plenty of exercise,
Such as biking, swimming, or going for a run;
Just get outside and be a kid;
Do lots of activities that you find fun!

It is important for your body to move;
Do not just stay inside and sit;
Grab some friends for a game of sports;
Together you can all stay fit!

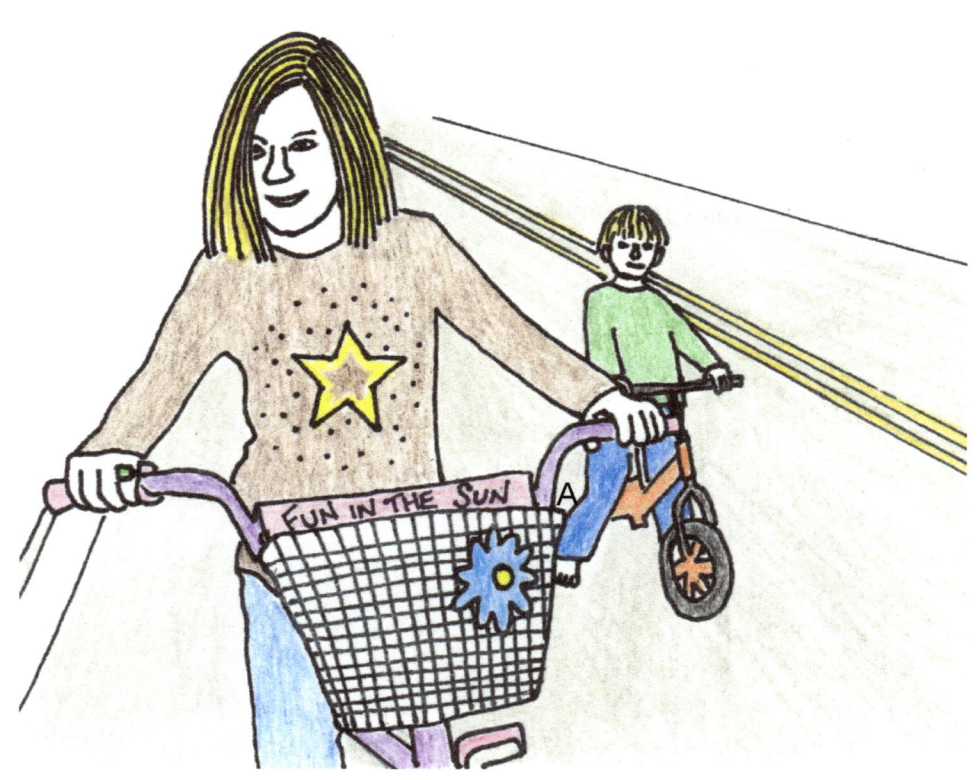

Unscramble these exercise activities:
(Answers on page 68)

kingih   _____

mmwiisng   _____

ccoers   _____

ginnnur   _____

sabellab   _____

kgiinb   _____

gksiin   _____

lllleybavo   _____

ckyeoh   _____

oobatfll   _____

katgsin   _____

ggiognj   _____

mpiungj oper   _____

xingob   _____

raatek   _____

ymnticssag   _____

fotalbls   _____

The Outdoorsy Stuff!

Vitamin D

Venture into the sunshine,
Just for a little bit each day;
So your body can produce Vitamin D,
From the sun's rays!

Although called a vitamin;
Technically it is not;
It is great for our overall health;
Just go for cover before you get too hot!

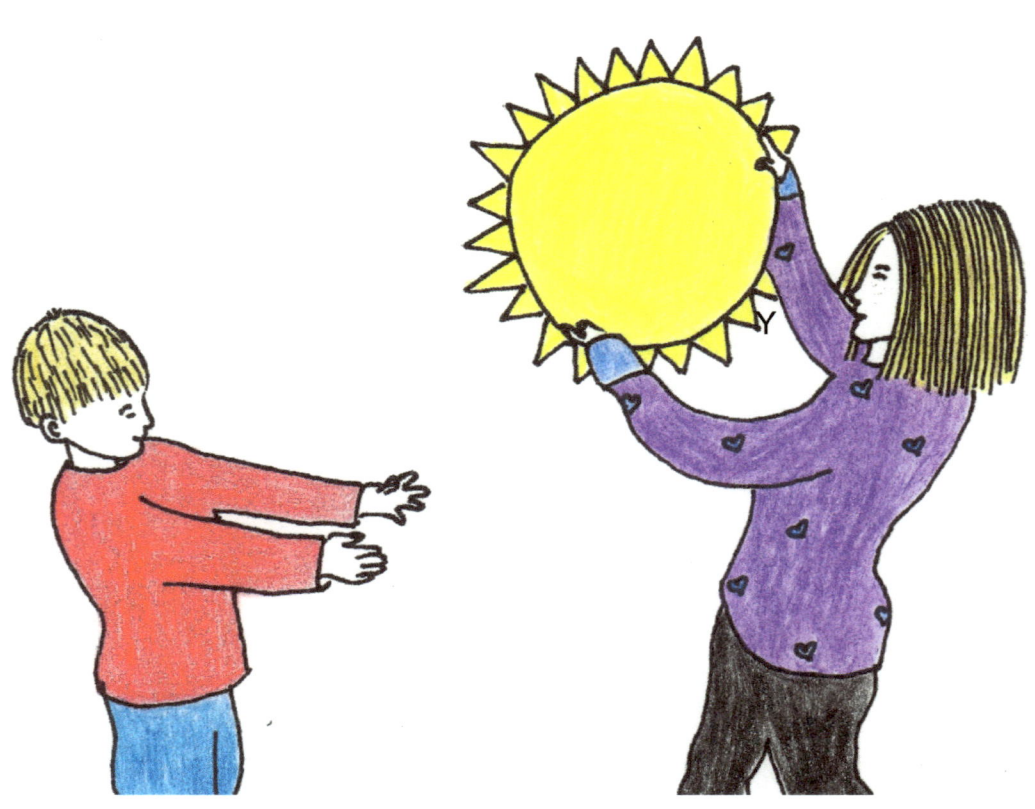

Definition:

Vitamin D-Can be produced by the body from sunlight and is super beneficial for overall health.

Challenge:
Enjoy the sunshine 10-20 minutes each day between 10:00am-2:00pm.

List your favorite things to do outside:

_____

_____

_____

_____

_____

_____

_____

_____

_____

_____

Nature

Get out in nature as much as you can;
Take a breath of fresh air and feel the breeze;
Run, play, and explore the land;
This is much healthier than watching TV!

Take a hike through the woods;
Look for creatures low and high;
Hear all the animals talk and sing;
Try counting the stars in the night sky!

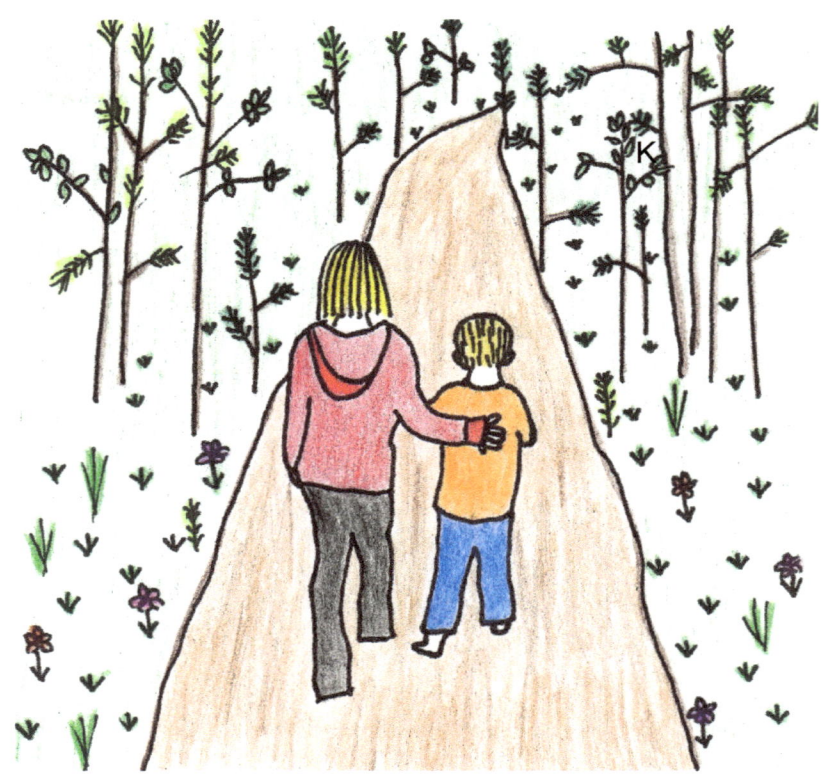

Challenge:

Go on a nature walk.

What cool things did you see?

_____

_____

_____

_____

_____

_____

_____

_____

_____

_____

Barefoot

Try to run around barefoot,
At every opportunity;
To absorb free electrons;
Earth's natural energy!

So kick off those shoes;
Run where the green grass grows;
Jump in a water puddle;
Feel the mud squish between your toes!

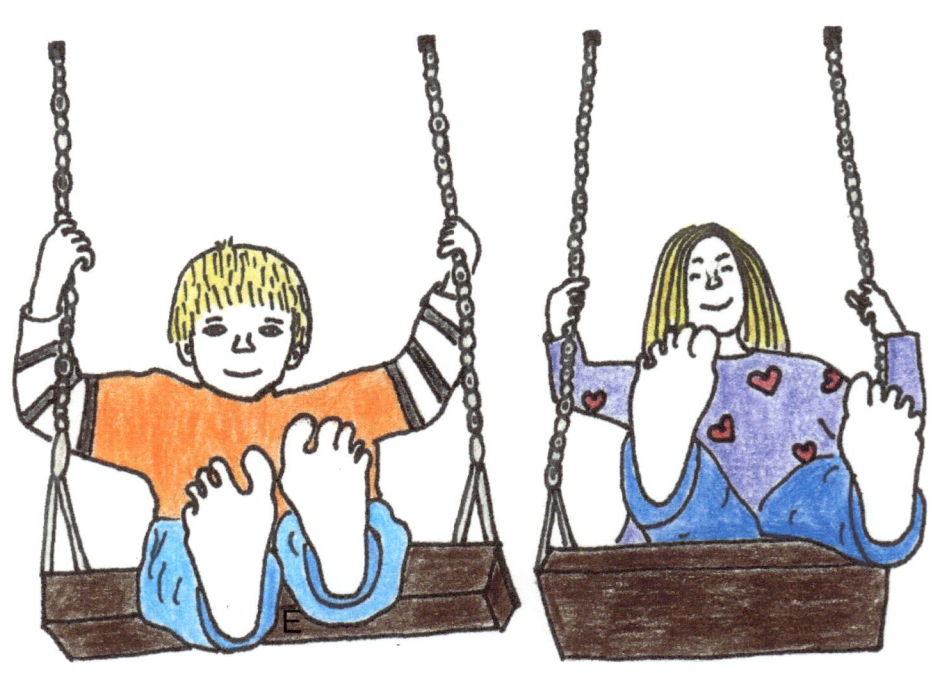

Definition:

Earthing/Grounding-Act of walking barefoot to absorb Earth's natural energy (electrons).

Challenge:

Walk barefoot!

Where did you walk barefoot?

_____

_____

_____

_____

_____

_____

_____

_____

_____

The Miscellaneous Stuff!

Sleep

It is important to get good quality sleep;
As a kid, eight to ten hours is best;
The earlier you go to bed;
The better your body can rest!

Try to get to bed at least by 9:00 o'clock;
Wind down in the evening with a calm activity;
Make sure your room is quiet and dark;
Don't fall asleep in front of the TV!

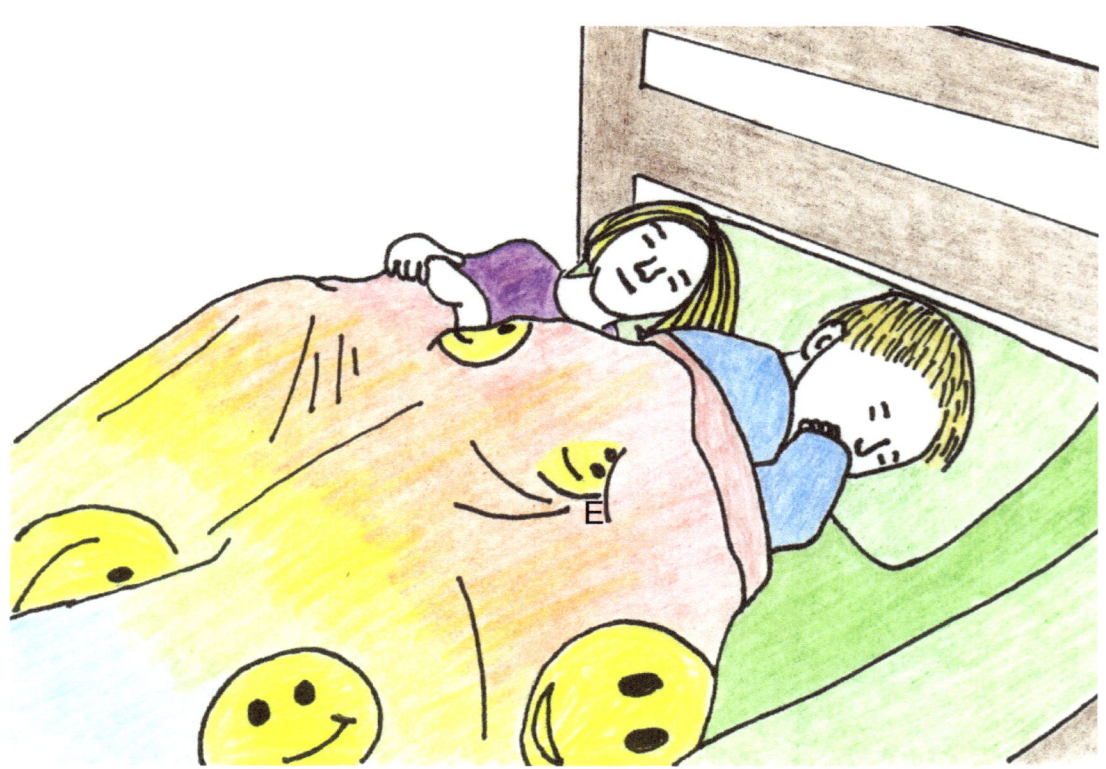

Sleep Facts:

1) Sleep is absolutely essential to good health. When sleeping, your brain recharges and your cells repair themselves.
2) Regular exercise normally improves your sleep. Just don't exercise right before bedtime.
3) Good sleep improves your memory and helps you live longer.
4) The stage of sleep called R.E.M. sleep stands for rapid eye movement. This is the stage of sleep in which most dreaming occurs.
5) Nightmares are just bad dreams that make you feel anxious or scared.

Sleep Fun Facts:

1) When whales & dolphins sleep, only half of their brain shuts down. The other half stays awake to help with breathing cycles.
2) One of the longest sleeping mammals is the Koala which sleeps about 22 hours a day.
3) Dreaming is normal. About 12% of people dream only in black and white.
4) It is impossible to sneeze while sleeping.
5) Sea otters hold hands when they are sleeping so they do not drift apart from each other.

Organization

It is good to be organized;
To have your stuff in order and neat;
If you take something out to use it,
Put it back when complete!

If your things are all over the place;
It creates such a mess;
Then when trying to find something;
It causes a lot more stress!

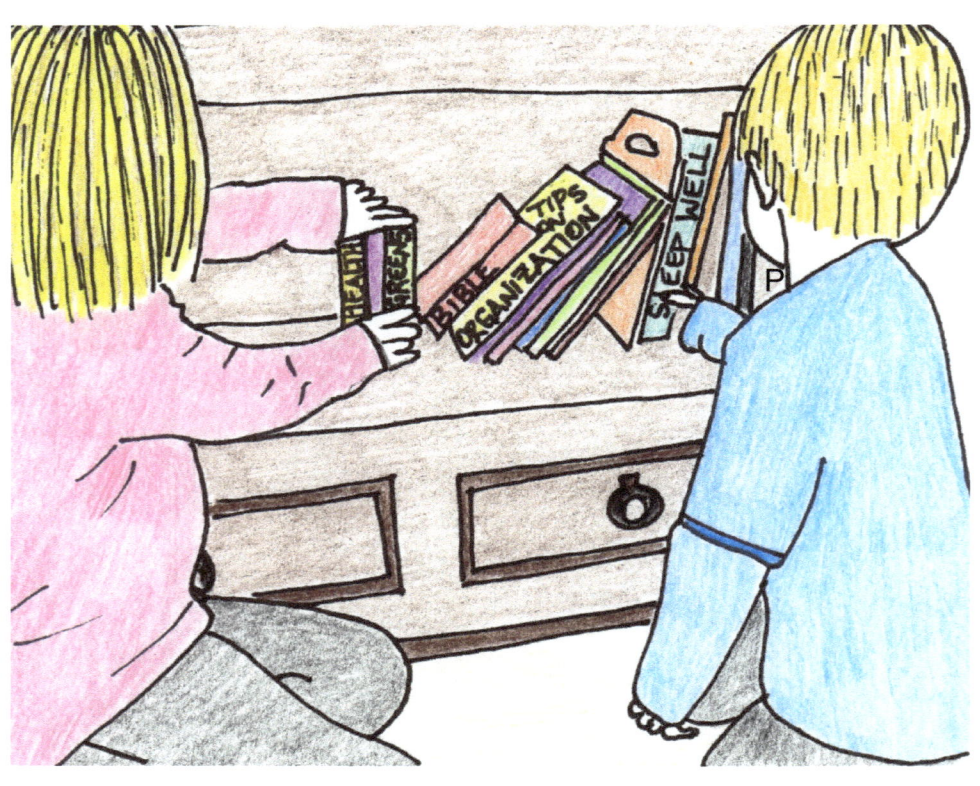

Definition:

Stress-a condition of being extremely anxious (worried).

Simple Organizational Tips:

1) Use containers to store things; especially smaller items.
2) Label storage containers to easily identify what is inside.
3) Sort and organize things by a common characteristic such as color, size, type, style, etc.
4) Frequently go through things and get rid of what is no longer necessary or being used.

Challenge:

Practice some of the organizational tips above.

Choices

Life is all about choices;
You can choose between good or bad;
You decide your own destiny;
Whether it is happy or sad!

For example, you can choose to be giving or greedy;
Healthy or unfit;
When life brings you lemons;
You can choose to be negative or positive about it!

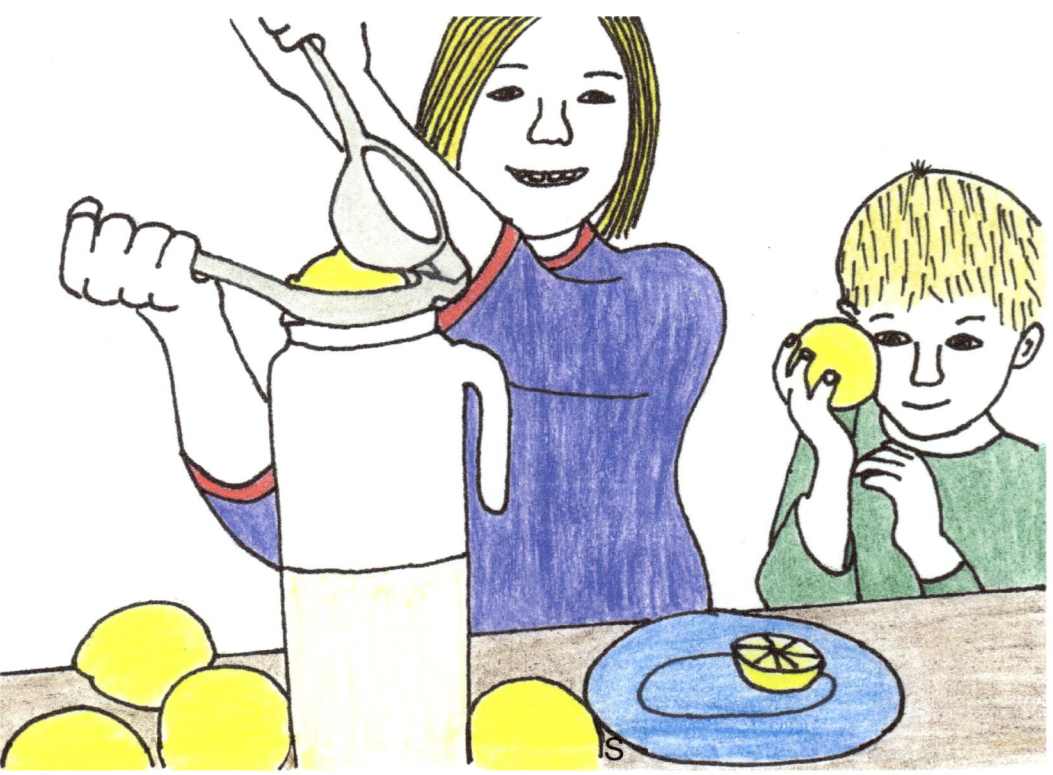

Cryptograms-Positive Choice Quotes:

Fill in the letters that correspond to the numbers below the blanks to solve the phrases and then write what you think they mean on the blank lines.
(Answers on page 68)

A	B	C	D	E	F	G	H	I	J	K	L	M	N	O	P	Q	R	S	T	U	V	W	X	Y	Z
6	24	19	23	5	8	4	17	18	12	2	3	14	13	26	21	9	11	10	25	20	7	22	15	1	16

"W H E N   L I F E   B R I N G S
 22 17 5 13   3 18 8 5   24 11 18 13 4 10

Y O U   L E M O N S;   M A K E
 1 26 20   3 5 14 26 13 10   14 6 2 5

L E M O N A D E!"
 3 5 14 26 13 6 23 5

_____

_____

_____

A	B	C	D	E	F	G	H	I	J	K	L	M	N	O	P	Q	R	S	T	U	V	W	X	Y	Z
6	24	19	23	5	8	4	17	18	12	2	3	14	13	26	21	9	11	10	25	20	7	22	15	1	16

"T A K E   T H E   H I G H   R O A D!"
 25 6 2 5   25 17 5   17 18 4 17   11 26 6 23

_____

_____

_____

Relationships (Friends)

When making friends,
Choose them with care;
Don't hang around bullies;
People who call names, tease, or pull other's hair!

Friends should be supportive;
Always willing to listen and be true;
They should lift your spirit up;
And like you for you!

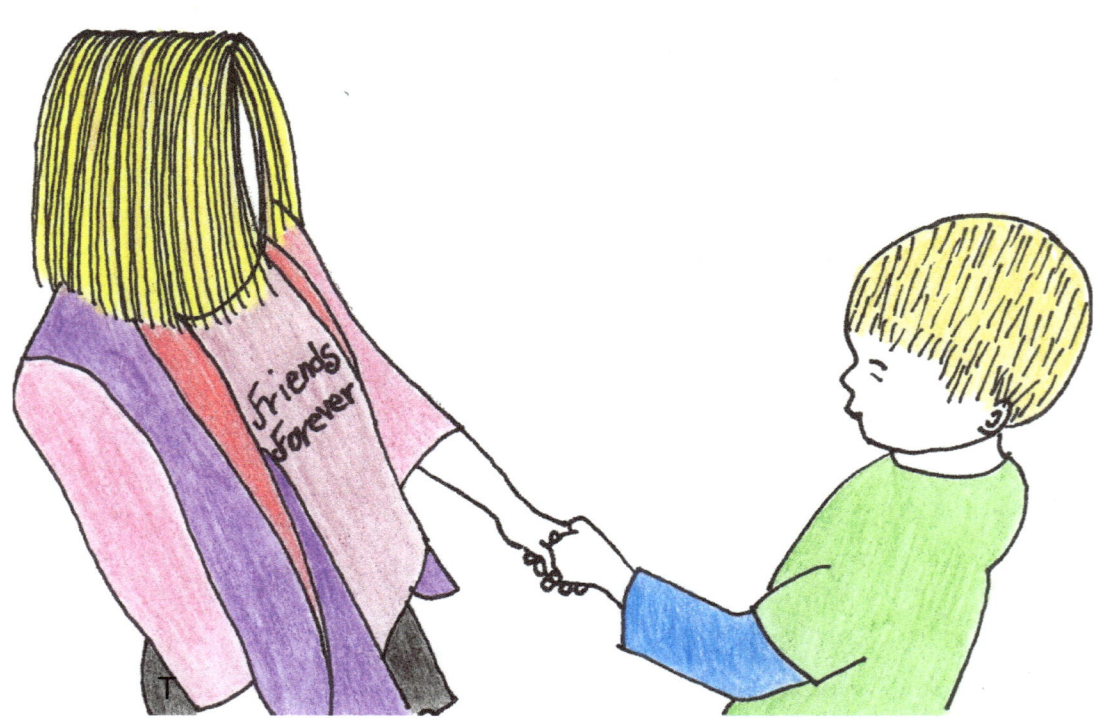

Challenge:

Who is a good friend?

_____.

What are some reasons you feel they are a good friend?

_____

_____

_____

_____

_____

Write a special thank you note to this person thanking them for being a good friend (Hint: You can include some of the reasons you listed above).

Hand Washing

Wash your hands throughout the day,
Especially before eating to stay healthy and clean;
Take your time to scrub a dub,
As you recite your ABCs or count some 123s!

Try not to worry so much about soap;
If so, use safe ones- preferably organic.
The rubbing and scrubbing causes friction,
Which is really what does the trick!

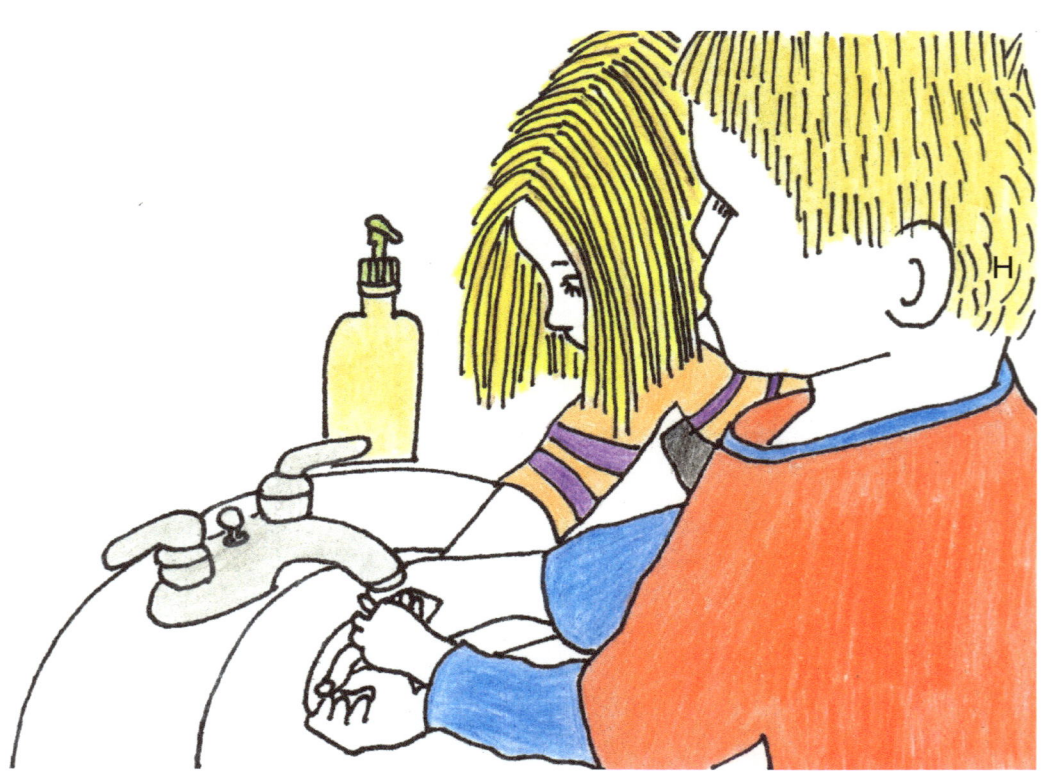

Definition:

Friction-the action of one surface or object rubbing against another.

The key (steps) to clean hands:

1) Wash frequently.
2) Warm water.
3) Soap-if safe, natural, organic.
4) Friction-rubbing and scrubbing.
5) Time-15 to 20 seconds.
6) Rinsing.

Challenge:

Practice the steps above to clean your hands.

What method do you use to make sure you wash your hands for at least 15-20 seconds?

a) I sing the ABC song.
b) I count.
c) I sing a different tune. If so, which one?

_____

d) Other. If so, what do you do?

_____

e) Nothing.

Plastic

Use as little plastic as possible;
It is not that reusable in the long-term;
It fills up the oceans and the landfills;
And is not safe if heated or if it burns!

Supposedly plastic numbered 1, 2, 4, or 5 is safe;
However, there is no guarantee on that deal;
It is best to use better alternatives;
Such as glass or stainless steel!

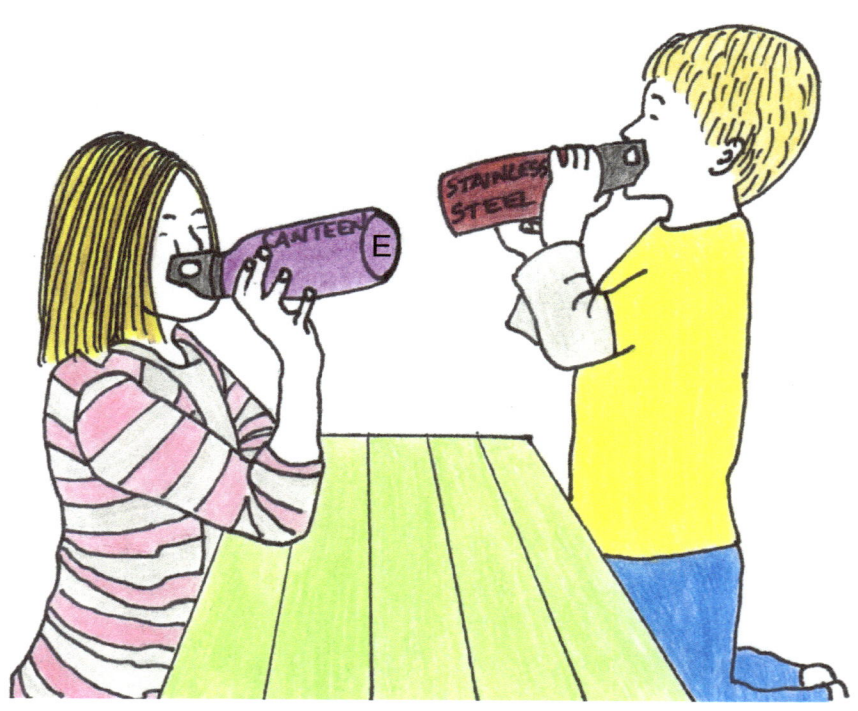

Use of plastic facts:

1) Fifty percent of the plastic used is only used once and then thrown away.
2) Enough plastic is thrown away to circle the Earth four times.
3) Plastic makes up about 90% of all the trash floating on the ocean's surface.
4) Every year lots of sea life die from eating plastic.

Challenges:

1) Ask for a safe, stainless steel (not aluminum) water bottle (canteen)...maybe as a birthday gift or at another gift getting opportunity!
2) If you are ever-so-lucky with challenge #1, don't leave home without it. Fill your canteen with water whenever you leave and forgo the plastic water bottles.
3) Please recycle plastic whenever possible if there is still a need to use it.

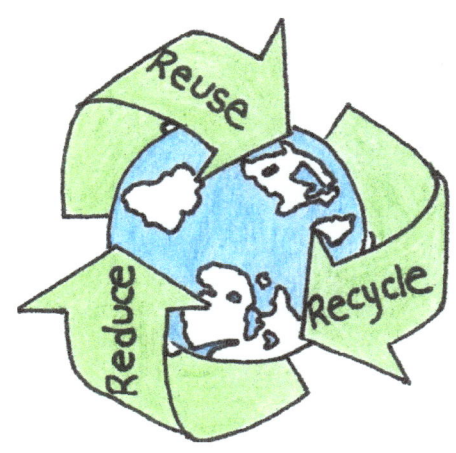

Chemicals (Scents)

Avoid a lot of smelly chemicals,
Found in lotions, perfumes, soaps, and shampoos;
Stuff that is scented with artificial fragrance;
That smells sweet, fruity, or flowery too!

It is bad for your body,
And not so good for your nose;
Over time you have to use more and more;
Because your sense of smell is hosed!

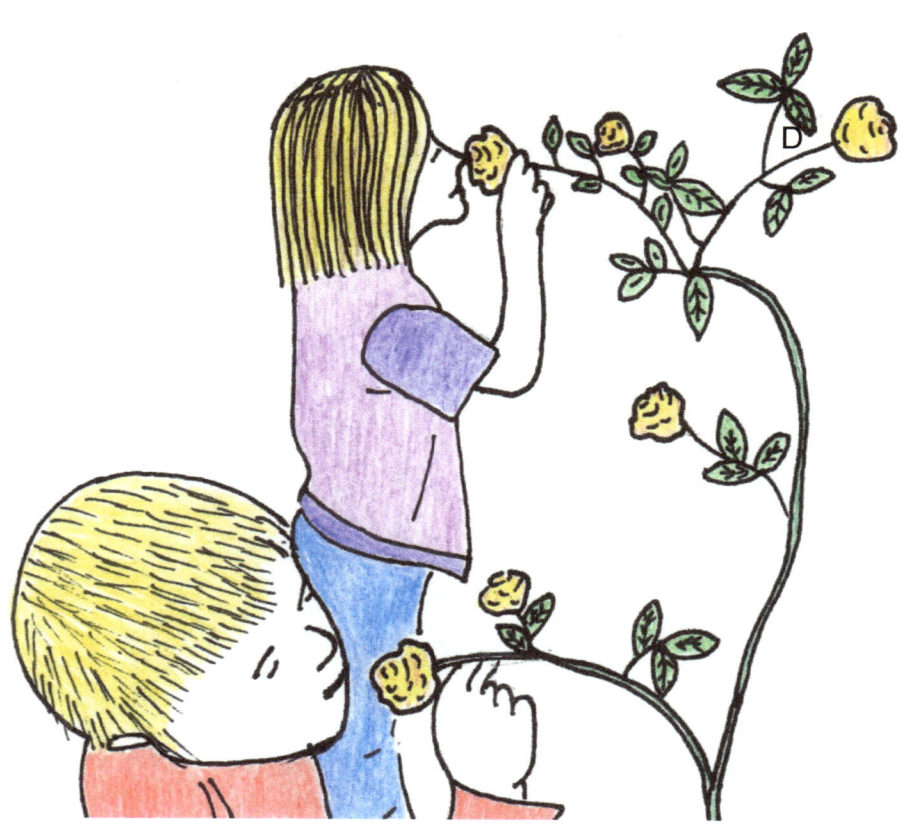

Definitions:

Fragrance-A sweet or delicate odor (smell).

Synthetic (artificial/not natural) fragrances-Ingredients derived from chemicals; known as petrochemicals. Synthetic fragrances are created in laboratories (labs).

Natural fragrances-Natural fragrances are essential oils and items derived from botanical (plant) ingredients that are harvested from the earth such as: flowers, fruits, sap, bark, leaves, and roots.

Hosed-'slang' (informal) term meaning attacked, assaulted, defeated. For example, the nose when it comes into contact with synthetic (artificial) smells.

Challenge:
Companies are allowed to use synthetic fragrances in products and just put the label 'fragrance' in the ingredients list. It is best to avoid products with the word 'fragrance'.

Look at your body care products (lotions, shampoos, etc.) and look for the word 'fragrance' in the ingredients list.

Which items did you find with the word 'fragrance'?

_____

_____

_____

Electronics

Limit electronics during the day;
Forgo the computers, phones, and TV;
Go outside to run, jump, and play;
Enjoy some physical activity!

Invite some friends over,
For an afternoon of games- old and new;
Be creative and imaginative;
Even invent some of your own too!

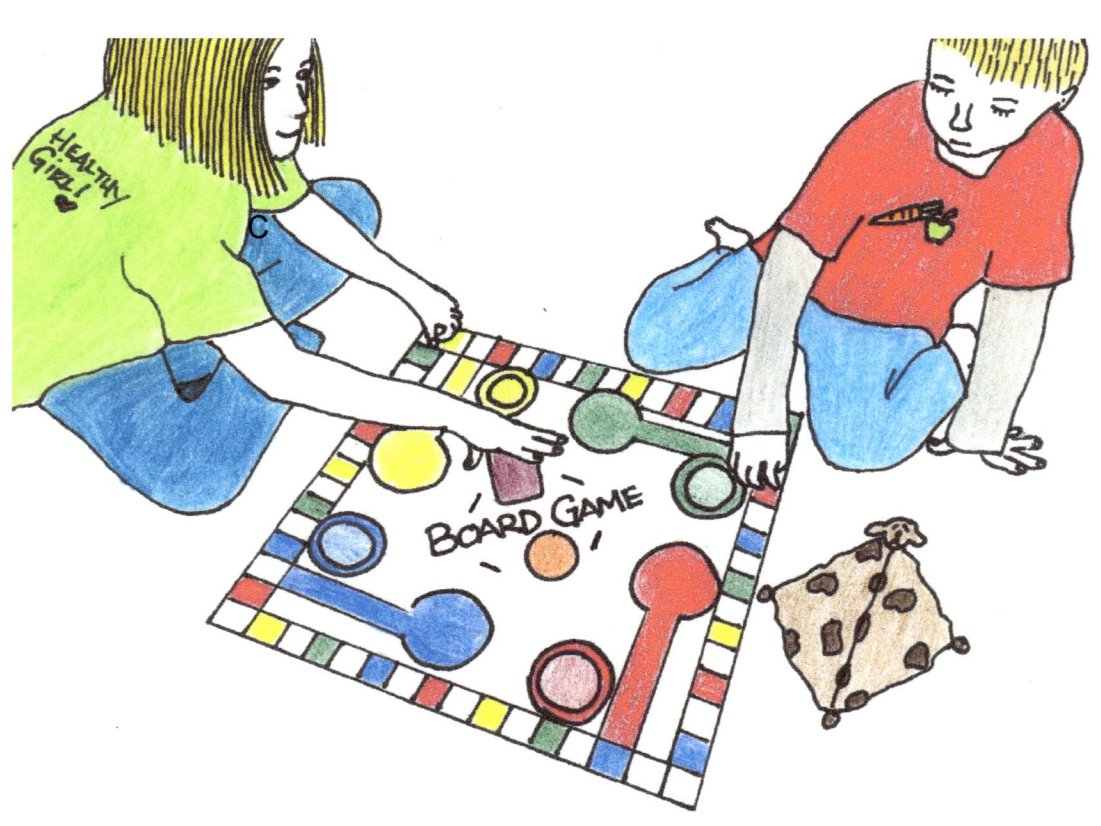

Challenge:
Limit/reduce the amount of time using electronics each day.

First, track the amount of time that you are using electronics daily for 3 days:

Day 1   Amount of time: _____

Day 2   Amount of time: _____

Day 3   Amount of time: _____

Average: Add the time from day 1, day 2, and day 3 and then divide by 3 (feel free to get help if needed).

Average amount of time each day: _____

Second, make a goal to reduce the average time calculated above. What is your goal: _____

What are some of your favorite non-electronic things to do?

_____

_____

_____

_____

What is your favorite game to play outside?

_____

What is your favorite board game to play?

_____

The Invaluable
Stuff!

<u>Invaluable</u>-having a worth so great that a value cannot be placed on it; priceless.

Positivity

Cut out the negativity,
In your words; with what you say;
Tell yourself positive things;
Like 'I matter' and 'I am loved today'!

Listen to happy music;
That fills your ears with uplifting words;
Steer clear of images of violence;
Which are bad for your thoughts and quite absurd!

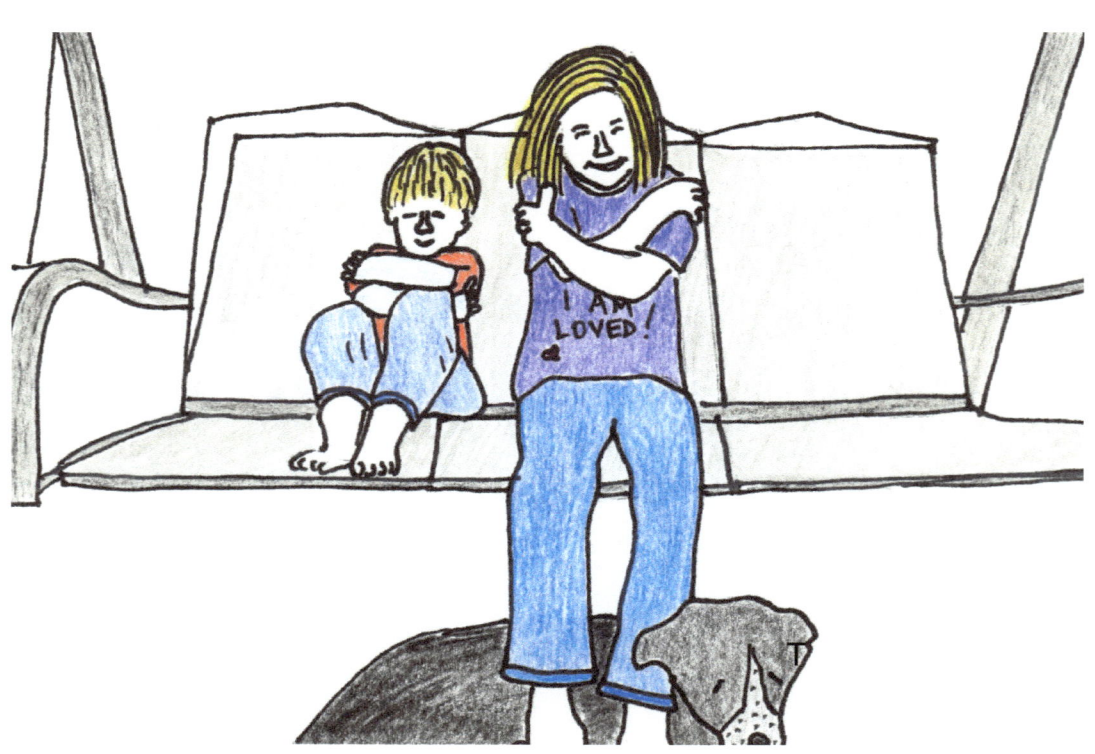

Challenge:

Look in the mirror and tell yourself something positive.

What did you tell yourself?

_____

Positive Quotes:

"Live life to the fullest, and focus on the positive."

Matt Cameron

"Always turn a negative situation into a positive situation."

Michael Jordan

"Delete the negative; accentuate the positive!"

Donna Karan

"You can't make positive choices for the rest of your life without an environment that makes those choices easy, natural, and enjoyable."

Deepak Chopra

"Choosing to be positive and having a grateful attitude is going to determine how you're going to live your life."

Joel Osteen

"Positive thinking will let you use the ability which you have, and that is awesome."

Zig Ziglar

Honesty

Speak your truth,
In a considerate way;
Don't tell lies;
Or people will lose confidence in what you say!

It is true that honesty,
Really is the best policy;
The more lies that are spoken;
The more you and others feel broken!

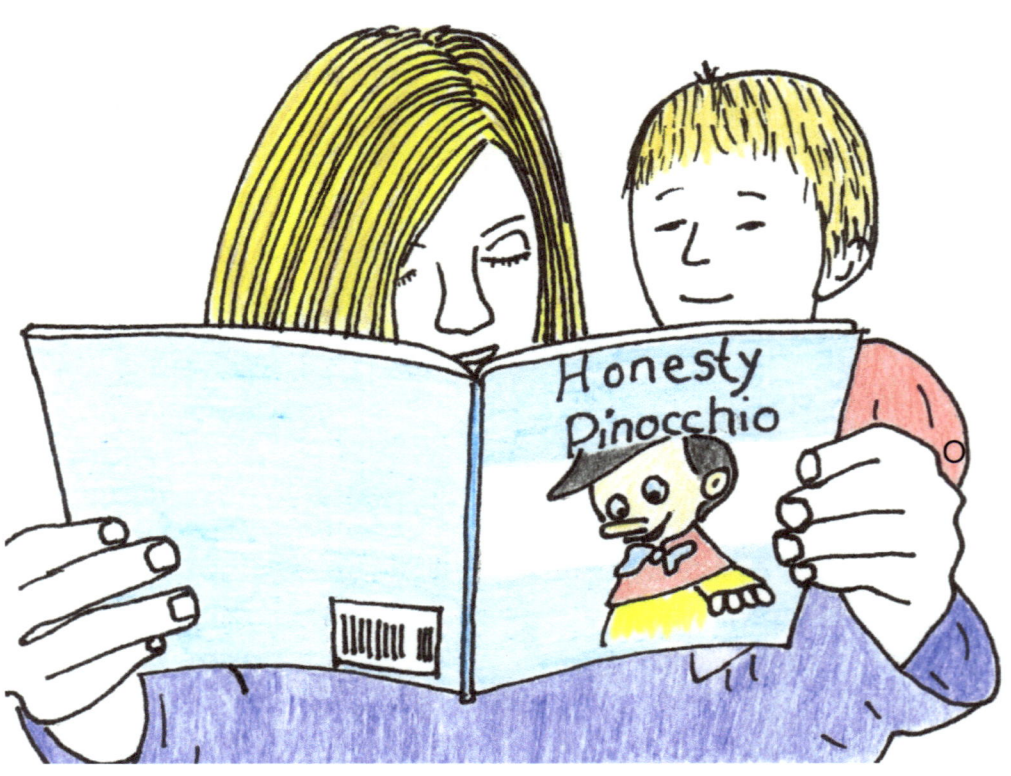

Challenge:

Write an apology letter to someone you told a lie to.

How many different words can you make from the letters in:

H   O   N   E   S   T   Y

_____

_____

_____

_____

_____

_____

_____

_____

_____

_____

_____

_____

Kindness

Practice grace and kindness,
All throughout your day;
Try to be helpful;
In your own way!

Do a good deed,
Just 'out of the blue';
You might just make someone's day;
It will make you feel good too!

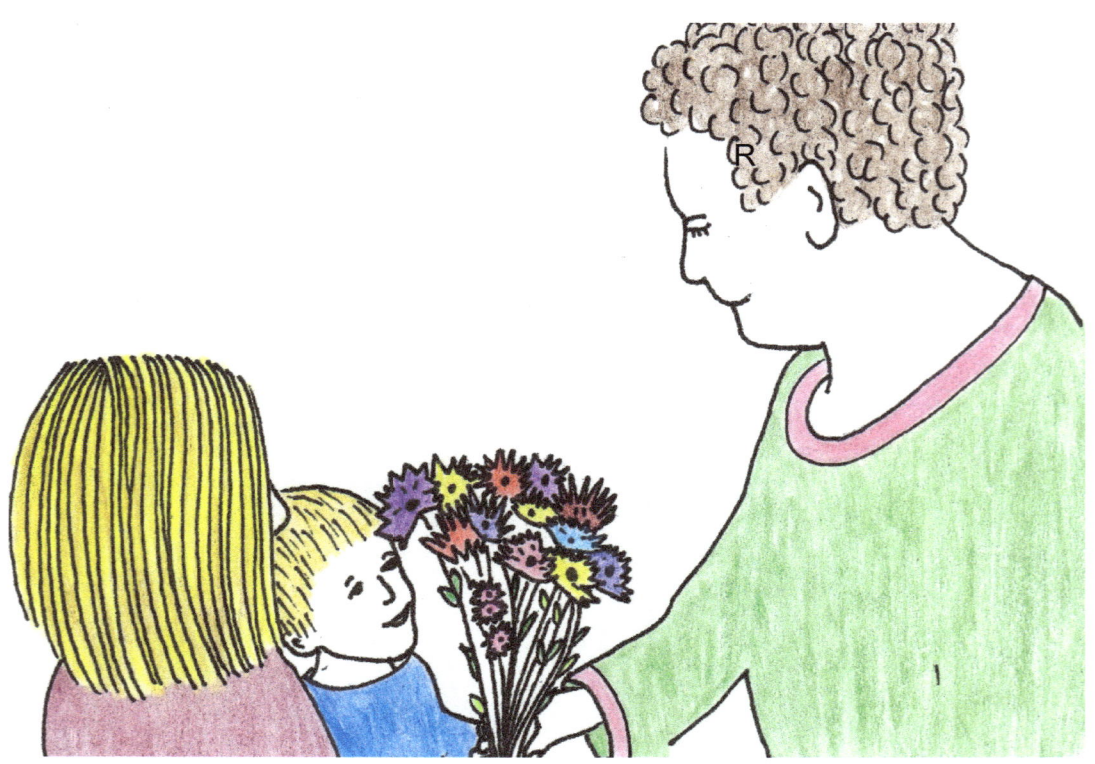

Challenge:

Do something nice for someone without them asking ('out of the blue').

What was your good deed?

_____

_____

How did it make you feel?

_____

_____

_____

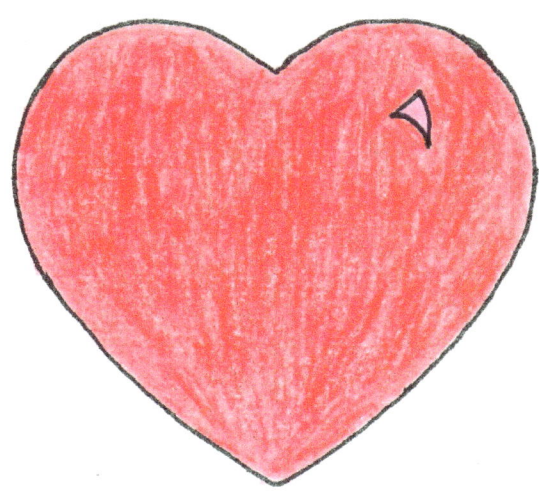

Gratitude

Be thankful whenever you can;
For all that comes your way;
Appreciate all that has happened;
Give thanks if not just a little bit each day!

Express gratitude for all the things in your life;
Include both big and small;
Show appreciation for people everywhere;
Being grateful is the best feeling of all!

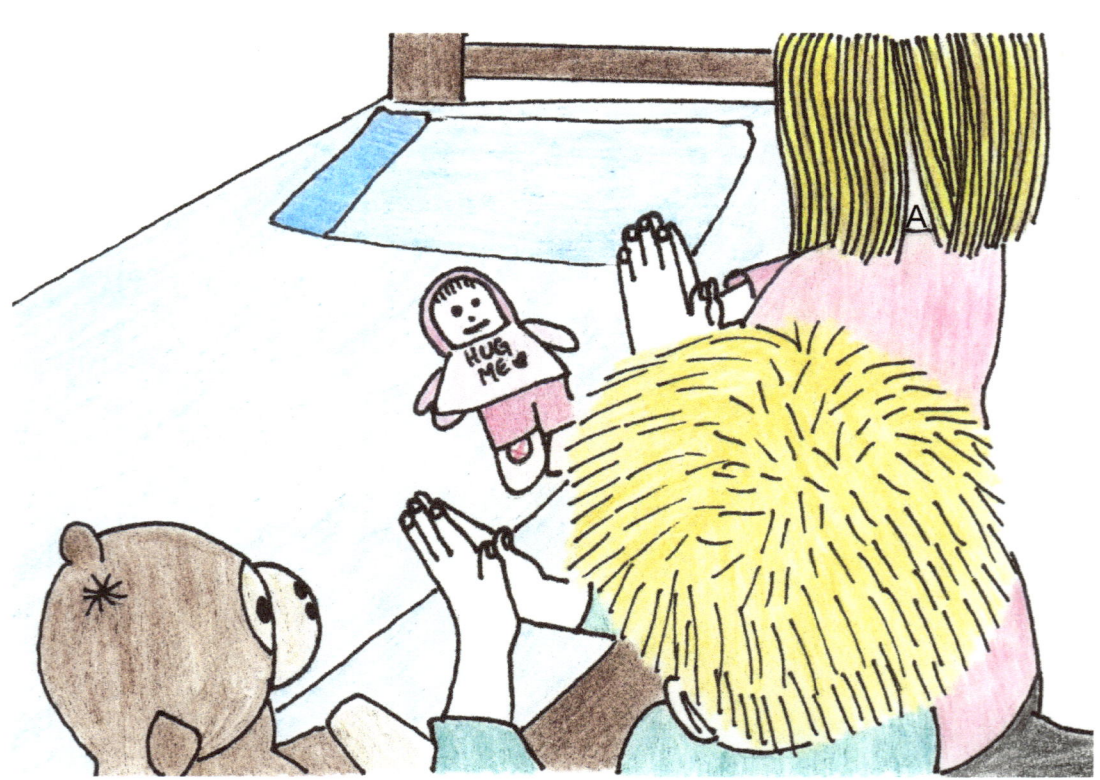

Challenge:

Keep a gratitude (thankfulness) journal for at least a week. Write down a few items you are grateful for each day.

Day	What are you thankful for?
Day 1	_____
Day 2	_____
Day 3	_____
Day 4	_____
Day 5	_____
Day 6	_____
Day 7	_____

Did you feel any different at the end of the week after showing gratitude? If so, how?

_____

_____

_____

Emotions (Feelings)

When it comes to emotions & feelings,
Most feel they have to keep them inside.
However, holding them in is not healthy;
Feel free to have a good cry!

Find someone you trust,
Like a parent, pastor, neighbor, or friend;
Someone you can express your feelings to;
Let it all out and you will feel better in the end!

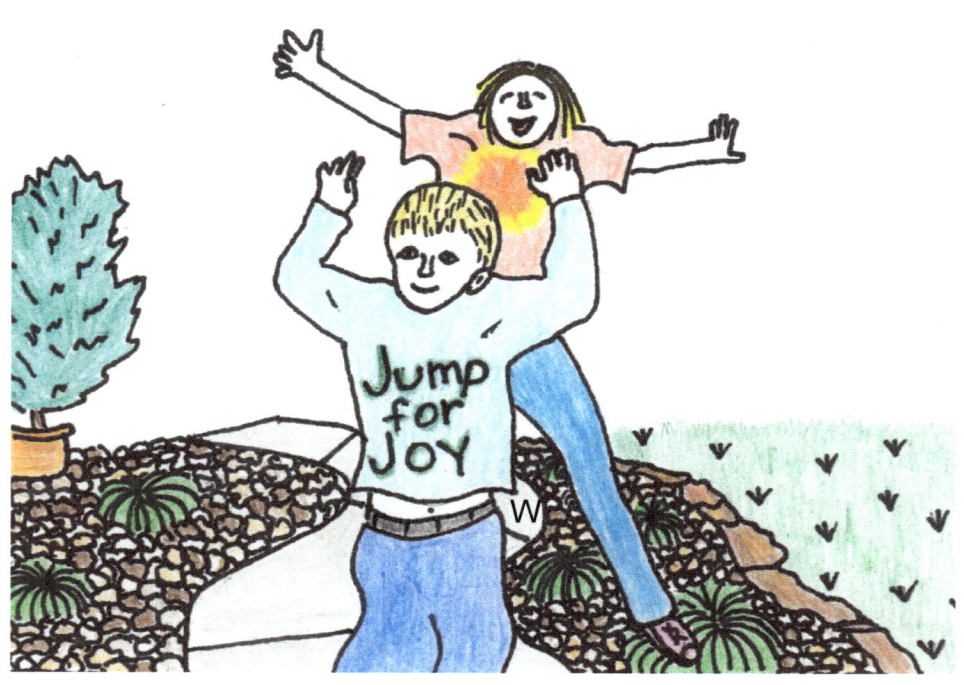

Definition:

Emotions (feelings)- a state of consciousness (awareness) in which joy, sadness, fear, anger, love, disgust, surprise, or the like is experienced.

Unscramble these emotions:
(Answers on page 68)

ovle   _____

geran   _____

ippessnha   _____

arfe   _____

yjo   _____

frsutratnio   _____

urprisse   _____

opeh   _____

mebarrassmnet _____

Who is someone you can trust to express your emotions (feelings) to?

_____

The Golden Rule

Treat people the way you want to be treated;
That is how the saying goes;
It's called 'The Golden Rule';
A great rule to live by to make friends- not foes!

If you want hugs, then give hugs;
If you want insults, then give insults;
Depending on how you treat others;
You can come to expect similar results!

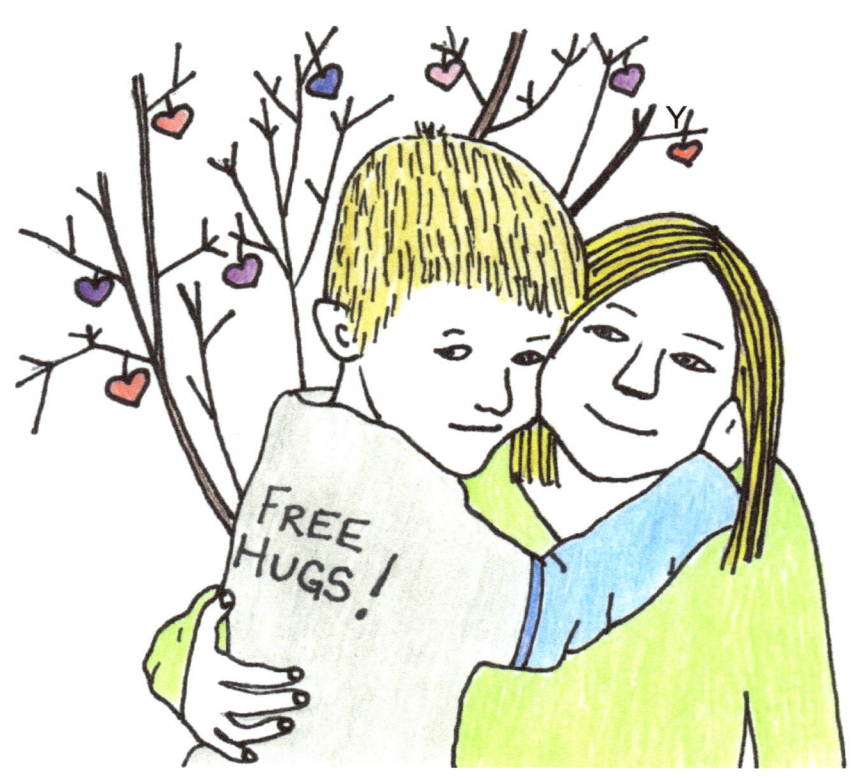

Fill in the letters that correspond to the numbers below
the blanks to solve this variation of The Golden Rule
(answer on page 68).

The Golden Rule

A B C D E F G H I J K L M N O P Q R S T U V W X Y Z
6 24 19 23 5 8 4 17 18 12 2 3 14 13 26 21 9 11 10 25 20 7 22 15 1 16

"
___ ___   ___ ___ ___ ___   ___ ___ ___ ___   ___ ___   ___ ___
23   26   20   13   25   26   26   25   17   5   11   10   6   10

___ ___ ___   ___ ___ ___ ___ ___   ___ ___ ___ ___
1   26   20   22   26   20   3   23   17   6   7   5

___ ___ ___ ___   ___ ___   ___ ___ ___ ___   ___   ___ ___ "
25   17   5   14   23   26   20   13   25   26   1   26   20

Luke 6:31

Secret Code

Each illustration within the topics has a hidden letter. Find the hidden letters and fill in the blanks below to decode the secret message!

The numbers below each blank are the page number where that letter can be found. Some letters are filled in for you!

The answer and more information are on page 68.

"__ __   __ __ P __ __   __   __ __ __
  8 10   12 14 16 18   20   22 24 28

__ __ __ __ __   __ __ __   __ O __ __ __ __
30 32 36 38 40   42 44 46   48   50 54 56 58

__ __ A __"
60 62   64

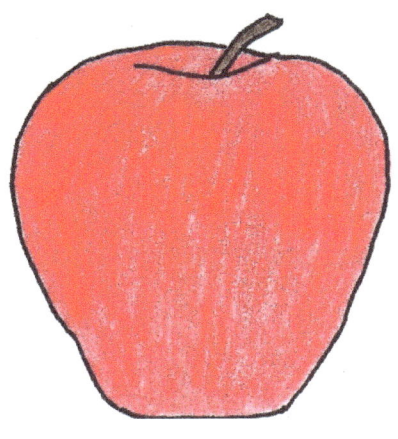

67

Answer Key

<u>Nutrition Labels (Ingredients)</u>:
Can you guess what food this is? Crunchy Cheetos

<u>Mindful Eating</u>:
True/False?:

  1) It is best to eat while watching a movie?   False
  2) When you are bored, it is best to grab a snack?   False
  3) It is best to eat because you are hungry?   True
  4) Chewing your food a lot is a waste of time?   False
  5) Eating until you are comfortably full is a good rule?   True

<u>Exercise</u>:
hiking, swimming, soccer, running, baseball, biking, skiing, volleyball, hockey, football, skating, jogging, jumping rope, boxing, karate, gymnastics, softball

<u>Choices</u>:

"When life brings you lemons; make lemonade." – to make the best out of a bad situation; to choose a positive action in the midst of something bad that has happened.

"Take the high road." – to choose to do the right thing in a situation even if it is hard and not what you really want to do.

<u>Emotions (Feelings)</u>:
love, anger, happiness, fear, joy, frustration, surprise, hope, embarrassment

<u>The Golden Rule</u>:
"Do unto others as you would have them do unto you"

<u>Secret Code</u>:
"An apple a day keeps the doctor away" is an old proverb (saying) which basically means eating healthy will keep you from going to the doctor.

Bibliography

Organic
1) "Organic Production/Organic Food: Information Access Tools", Compiled by Mary V Gold June 2007, Accessed February 2015, http://www.nal.usda.gov/afsic/pubs/ofp/ofp.shtml
2) "Locally Grown", by Jennifer Chait, accessed February 2015, http://organic.about.com/od/organicdefinitionskl/g/Locally-Grown.htm
3) "Local & Regional Food Systems", Grace Communications Foundation, accessed February 2015, http://www.sustainabletable.org/254/local-regional-food-systems
4) "What is the difference between organic and conventional food?", European Food Information Council, accessed February 2015, http://www.eufic.org/page/en/page/FAQ/faqid/difference-organic-conventional-food/
5) "Definition of Conventional and Organic Food", Answers, accessed February 2015, http://nutrition.answers.com/healthy-foods/definition-of-conventional-and-organic-food
6) "Top 10 Most Common GMO Foods", Eat Local Grown, accessed February 2015, http://eatlocalgrown.com/article/12060-top-gmo-foods.html
7) "What is GMO?", Non-GMO Project, accessed February 2015, http://www.nongmoproject.org/learn-more/what-is-gmo/
8) "What Do Those Codes On Stickers Of Fruits And Some Veggies Mean?", Dr. Frank Lipman, November 2002, accessed February 2015, http://www.drfranklipman.com/what-do-those-codes-on-stickers-of-fruits-and-some-veggies-mean/

Fruits
1) "Fruit or vegetable-Do you know the difference?", By Jennifer K. Nelson, R.D., L.D. and Katherine Zeratsky, R.D., L.D. August 15, 2012, accessed February 2015, http://www.mayoclinic.org/healthy-living/nutrition-and-healthy-eating/expert-blog/fruit-vegetable-difference/bgp-20056141

Water
1) "20 Interesting and Useful Water Facts", AllAboutWater.org, accessed February 2015, http://www.allaboutwater.org/water-facts.html
2) "Water Facts", Science and Kids, accessed February 2015, http://www.sciencekids.co.nz/sciencefacts/water.html
3) "Water: How much should you drink every day?", Mayo Clinic Staff, accessed February 2015, http://www.mayoclinic.org/healthy-living/nutrition-and-healthy-eating/in-depth/water/art-20044256

Sugar
1) "14 Mind-Blowing Facts About Sugar (Infographic)", by Jason Wachob, April 16, 2012, accessed February 2015, http://www.mindbodygreen.com/0-4543/14-MindBlowing-Facts-About-Sugar-Infographic.html
2) The Free Dictionary by Farlex, accessed February 2015, http://www.thefreedictionary.com/addicting

Nutrition Labels
1) Frito Lay website, accessed March 6, 2015, http://www.fritolay.com/snacks/product-page/cheetos/cheetos-crunchy-cheese-flavored-snacks

Mindful Eating
1) "What is Mindful Eating?", Am I Hungry?, accessed February 2015, http://amihungry.com/what-is-mindful-eating/

Macronutrients
1) "Macronutrients: the Importance of Carbohydrate, Protein, and Fat", McKinley Health Center, accessed February 2015, http://www.mckinley.illinois.edu/handouts/macronutrients.htm

Vitamin D
1) "what are the health benefits of vitamin D?", Medical News Today, Last updated: Friday 6 February 2015, accessed February 2015, http://www.medicalnewstoday.com/articles/161618.php

Barefoot
1) "The Ultimate Antioxidant: Fight Premature Aging for Free", Mercola.com, November 4, 2012, accessed February 2015, http://articles.mercola.com/sites/articles/archive/2012/11/04/why-does-walking-barefoot-on-the-earth-make-you-feel-better.aspx

Sleep
1) "25 Random Facts about Sleep", National Sleep Foundation, accessed February 2015, http://sleepfoundation.org/sleep-news/25-random-facts-about-sleep
2) "16 Amazing Facts About Sleep That Will Surely Impress You", Anna Chui, accessed February 2015, http://www.lifehack.org/articles/lifestyle/16-amazing-facts-about-sleep-that-will-surely-impress-you.html

Organization
1) Merriam-Webster, accessed February 2015, http://www.merriam-webster.com/dictionary/stress

Hand Washing
1) Merriam-Webster, accessed February 2015, http://www.merriam-webster.com/dictionary/friction

Bibliography Continued

Plastic
1) "22 Facts About Plastic Pollution (And 10 Things We Can Do About It)", Lynn Hasselberger, April 17, 2014, accessed February 2015, http://ecowatch.com/2014/04/07/22-facts-plastic-pollution-10-things-can-do-about-it/
2) "The Numbers on Plastic Bottles: What do Plastic Recycling Symbols Mean?", Mike Barrett, Wednesday 6 February 2013, accessed February 2015, http://www.nationofchange.org/numbers-plastic-bottles-what-do-plastic-recycling-symbols-mean-1360168347

Chemicals (Scents)
1) Merriam-Webster, accessed February 2015, http://www.merriam-webster.com/dictionary/fragrance
2) "Natural Perfume vs. Synthetic Perfume", Pour le Monde, accessed February 2015, http://www.pourlemondeparfums.com/naturalvssynthetic.html

Invaluable
1) Merriam-Webster, accessed February 2015, http://www.merriam-webster.com/dictionary/invaluable

Emotions/Feelings
1) Merriam-Webster, accessed February 2015, http://www.merriam-webster.com/dictionary/emotions

Puzzles
Terms of Use Policy

Our copyright notice applies to our Online Puzzle Maker.

As for the puzzles you create with our Online Puzzle Maker, you are free to use them in any way you wish, even commercially. Please give credit (e.g., "Puzzle made at puzzle-maker.com").

As a condition of using this online puzzle maker, your words and clues will help build a database of words and clues that will help other teachers and puzzle makers in the future. We might also be retaining, editing and reusing certain puzzles that are particularly well done.